T0365318

Cambridge Elements ≡

Elements of Improving Quality and Safety in Healthcare
edited by
Mary Dixon-Woods,* Katrina Brown,* Sonja Marjanovic,†
Tom Ling,† Ellen Perry,* Graham Martin,* Gemma Petley,* and
Claire Dipple*
*THIS Institute (The Healthcare Improvement Studies Institute)
†RAND Europe

MEASUREMENT FOR IMPROVEMENT

Alene Toulany[1,2] and Kaveh G. Shojania[2,3]
[1] The Hospital for Sick Children (SickKids), Toronto,
Ontario, Canada
[2] Faculty of Medicine, University of Toronto, Canada
[3] Sunnybrook Health Sciences Centre, Toronto,
Ontario, Canada

THIS.Institute The Healthcare Improvement Studies Institute

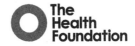

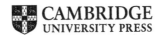

CAMBRIDGE
UNIVERSITY PRESS

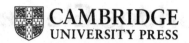

Shaftesbury Road, Cambridge CB2 8EA, United Kingdom

One Liberty Plaza, 20th Floor, New York, NY 10006, USA

477 Williamstown Road, Port Melbourne, VIC 3207, Australia

314–321, 3rd Floor, Plot 3, Splendor Forum, Jasola District Centre, New Delhi – 110025, India

103 Penang Road, #05–06/07, Visioncrest Commercial, Singapore 238467

Cambridge University Press is part of Cambridge University Press & Assessment, a department of the University of Cambridge.

We share the University's mission to contribute to society through the pursuit of education, learning and research at the highest international levels of excellence.

www.cambridge.org
Information on this title: www.cambridge.org/9781009326056

DOI: 10.1017/9781009326063

First published 2025

A catalogue record for this publication is available from the British Library

ISBN 978-1-009-32605-6 Paperback
ISSN 2754-2912 (online)
ISSN 2754-2904 (print)

Cambridge University Press & Assessment has no responsibility for the persistence or accuracy of URLs for external or third-party internet websites referred to in this publication and does not guarantee that any content on such websites is, or will remain, accurate or appropriate.

Every effort has been made in preparing this Element to provide accurate and up-to-date information that is in accord with accepted standards and practice at the time of publication. Although case histories are drawn from actual cases, every effort has been made to disguise the identities of the individuals involved. Nevertheless, the authors, editors, and publishers can make no warranties that the information contained herein is totally free from error, not least because clinical standards are constantly changing through research and regulation. The authors, editors, and publishers therefore disclaim all liability for direct or consequential damages resulting from the use of material contained in this Element. Readers are strongly advised to pay careful attention to information provided by the manufacturer of any drugs or equipment that they plan to use.

Measurement for Improvement

Elements of Improving Quality and Safety in Healthcare

DOI: 10.1017/9781009326063
First published online: January 2025

Alene Toulany[1,2] and Kaveh G. Shojania[2,3]
[1] *The Hospital for Sick Children (SickKids), Toronto, Ontario, Canada*
[2] *Faculty of Medicine, University of Toronto, Canada*
[3] *Sunnybrook Health Sciences Centre, Toronto, Ontario, Canada*

Author for correspondence: Kaveh G. Shojania,
kaveh.shojania@sunnybrook.ca

Abstract: The main principles underpinning measurement for healthcare improvement are outlined in this Element. Although there is no single formula for achieving optimal measurement to support improvement, a fundamental principle is the importance of using multiple measures and approaches to gathering data. Using a single measure falls short in capturing the multifaceted aspects of care across diverse patient populations, as well as all the intended and unintended consequences of improvement interventions within various quality domains. Even within a single domain, improvement efforts can succeed in several ways and go wrong in others. Therefore, a family of measures is usually necessary. Clearly communicating a plausible theory outlining how an intervention will lead to desired outcomes informs decisions about the scope and types of measurement used. Improvement teams must tread carefully to avoid imposing undue burdens on patients, clinicians, or organisations. This title is also available as Open Access on Cambridge Core.

Keywords: measurement, family of measures, bias, stakeholder engagement, validity

ISBNs: 9781009326056 (PB), 9781009326063 (OC)
ISSNs: 2754-2912 (online), 2754-2904 (print)

Contents

1 Introduction

Measurement is a key characteristic of any healthcare improvement effort. 'If you can't measure it, you can't improve it', is a widely quoted mantra, often attributed to engineer, statistician, and management pioneer Edwards Deming. It is true that Deming saw measurement as fundamental to improvement work. But what he actually said is rather different: 'It is wrong to suppose that if you can't measure it, you can't manage it – a costly myth'.[1,2] Deming recognised that management can occur on the basis of what we might now call qualitative signals or 'soft intelligence'.[3,4] In practice, most improvement interventions benefit from a mix of qualitative and quantitative measures – certainly during the development and refinement of an intervention and often in its eventual evaluation.

In this Element, we outline the major principles that underpin measurement related to healthcare improvement. We cover core concepts relevant to any measure (e.g. content and construct validity) and identify some unique problems that arise specifically in the context of measurement for improvement.

Although there is no single formula to guide us in how best to use measurement to support improvement, the importance of using multiple measures is crucial. Any improvement effort can succeed in several ways and go wrong in others. Moreover, contemporary definitions of quality identify distinct domains, including safety, effectiveness, patient-centredness, equity, and efficiency. No single measure (or probably even no measurement approach) can capture all the relevant intended and unintended consequences from any given intervention across multiple domains. Properly evaluating any improvement intervention usually needs a family of measures to overcome these challenges.

2 Measuring Healthcare Quality

The triad of structure, process, and outcome was first articulated by Avedis Donabedian in the 1960s,[5–8] and it remains the predominant model underpinning measurement of healthcare quality. Outcomes – from morbidity and mortality to functional status and the patient experience – are the bottom line for quality measurement. But outcomes are also a challenge for measurement. Mortality is easy to measure but doesn't represent the main outcome of interest for most improvement interventions. Harms short of death (i.e. morbidity) are more often relevant, but determining how many patients avoid key complications or achieve important functional outcomes is often far from straightforward.

2.1 Structural Measures

Donabedian pointed out that when connections exist between structural elements of care and patient outcomes of interest, it is possible to focus on the structural elements as they are often relatively easy to measure. For instance, an extensive literature shows associations between patient volume (i.e. the number of patients treated) and improved outcomes,[9] especially for surgical procedures.[10,11] Rather than measuring multiple outcomes after surgery, one might simply assess surgical volumes – as one prominent healthcare coalition in the United States has done.[12]

But this example highlights both the promise and potential pitfalls of structural measures: although they can be easy to measure and are usually easily understood by decision-makers and members of the public (e.g. 'practice makes perfect' for surgical volumes), structural aspects of care can be hard to change – and the benefits of doing so are far from guaranteed. Suppose, for example, that one hospital in a region becomes designated as the only one to perform certain complex cancer surgeries. It's not guaranteed that a several-fold increase in the number of patients at that hospital will immediately reproduce the good outcomes of centres that have performed this procedure at high volumes for many years. A rapid increase in patient volumes might even worsen care.

Also, the supporting evidence for most structural measures comes from observational studies potentially influenced by other factors. For instance, a substantial literature documents lower morbidity and mortality in hospitals where fewer patients are cared for by each nurse.[13,14] Such a relationship is extremely plausible, but it is also plausible that hospitals with better staffing levels are doing other things that are also conducive to improved patient outcomes.

2.2 Process Measures

Instead of depicting hospitals and clinics as black boxes with broad structural features, process measures take us inside the black box to capture the care patients actually receive. Process measures can include education and counselling (e.g. smoking cessation, encouraging physical activity), preventive care (e.g. age-appropriate vaccines, cancer screening), and provision of established medicines and surgeries. How these aspects of care are delivered can also count as process measures (Box 1).

One disadvantage of process measures, however, is that they are understood primarily by clinicians. The percentages of patients who received x, y, and z medicines or had a door-to-balloon time under 90 minutes have no obvious messages for patients. Table 1 lists commonly cited advantages and disadvantages

Box 1 PROCESS MEASURES RELATED TO CARE DELIVERY

A large body of evidence shows that for patients with acute ST-elevation myocardial infarction (a heart attack with a completely blocked coronary artery), the best outcomes occur when the time from hospital arrival to performance of percutaneous coronary intervention (a procedure to open up blood vessels in the heart) does not exceed 90 minutes.[15] Similar evidence exists for thrombolysis for acute stroke, and as a result 'door-to-needle' time has become a common process-based target in efforts to improve the quality of acute stroke care.[16]

Delivering a given treatment can itself count as a process measure and so can the way it is delivered (e.g. its timeliness). A benefit of using process measures is that they identify targets for improvement more directly than outcome measures do, and they can do so fairly quickly. It might take years to see quality differences between hospitals using risk-adjusted (accounting for individual patient risk factors) mortality for patients with acute myocardial infarction; significant differences in the percentage of patients who receive recommended processes of care can become apparent within months.[17]

A hospital with a higher than expected 30-day mortality among patients with acute myocardial infarction will need to examine numerous potential contributing factors. But a hospital with prolonged door-to-balloon time – the time from arrival at the hospital to the patient undergoing the cardiac catheterisation procedure – will be clearer about where it needs to focus. Yet, processes of care themselves depend on multiple other processes. The hospital wanting to lower its door-to-balloon time needs to consider what paramedics do for patients in the field, aspects of care in the emergency department, how the cardiology team is activated, and so on.[18]

of process measures, though some do not withstand close scrutiny. For instance, outcome-based measures notoriously run into debates over the adequacy of adjustment for casemix – referring to the mix of patient characteristics and conditions that can influence outcomes. Process measures supposedly avoid that problem, but a similar problem can sneak in due to differences in potential exceptions or contraindications. For example, general practices judged on their rates of childhood vaccination might have different proportions of parents who choose for their child not to receive vaccines.

In addition, processes of care as measured may not capture the reality of process delivery. For instance, a typical note in a patient's medical record might mention 'patient counselled on smoking cessation'. A clinic could score very

Table 1 The triad of structure, process, and outcome for measuring healthcare quality

Approaches to assessment	Definition	Examples*	Advantages	Disadvantages
Structure	Attributes of the settings in which care occurs – e.g. infrastructure, human resources, availability of specific technologies and services, models of care, and organisational culture, among others.	Hospital size, teaching status, ownership. Availability of specific technologies and services. Staffing ratios and skill mix. Patient volumes. Clinical information systems. Organisational culture. Models of care (e.g. stroke units, closed intensive care units).	Efficient measurement. Captures aspects of care with the potential to affect multiple processes and outcomes of care.	Blunt. Often hard to change. Not always clear if change will produce improvement.
Process	The actions involved in delivering care, including those relating to screening, diagnosing, and treating.	Percentage of patients undergoing evidence-based cancer screening. Provision of proven medicines for patients with	Directly measures the care patients receive. Detects likely quality problems without having to	Often has little meaning for patients or decision-makers.

	Definition	Examples	Strengths	Limitations/Challenges
		acute myocardial infarction. Venous thromboembolism for hospitalised patients. Appropriate screening for retinal disease in patients with diabetes. Discussion of advanced directives and goals of care. Informed consent.	wait for poor outcomes to become apparent. Less sensitive to casemix differences than outcome measures. Directly suggests targets for healthcare improvement.	Accounting for legitimate exceptions can be deceptively challenging. Documentation not necessarily tied to the real process of interest (e.g. medical records document the prescriptions of interest, but there is no guarantee patients took the medicines as intended). Identification of targets for improvement not as straightforward as may appear (see text).
Outcome	Effects of care on the health status of patients and populations.	Mortality. Complications/morbidity. Patient Reported Outcome Measures (PROMs).	Meaningful to patients, providers, and decision-makers. Captures ultimate goal of measurement and improvement efforts.	Multiple factors influence outcomes. Adjustment for differences in casemix often challenging.

Table 1 (cont.)

Approaches to assessment	Definition	Examples*	Advantages	Disadvantages
		Patient Reported Experience Measures (PREMs). Hospital Consumer Assessment of Healthcare Providers and Systems (HCAHPS).		Often require long observation periods to detect problems.

*The examples in Table 1 have been chosen for illustrative purposes on the basis of having been used as structural measures or their potential indicated for such use in the literature. This should not be taken as indicating a justified, well-established use in performance measurement.

well on the percentage of patients with such notes in their records, no matter how brief the advice given was, or how far removed from the intense support given in the trials that established smoking cessation counselling as a process-based quality measure in the first place. The same applies for more straightforward processes, such as medicine prescriptions: a clinic could prescribe recommended inhalers to most asthma patients, yet patients might not be using them in the recommended manner.

2.3 Outcome Measures

Outcome measures have the advantage of holding meaning from all points of view: patients, commissioners, and healthcare professionals. Yet outcomes also reflect factors other than the quality of care, including how sick the patient is, socioeconomic determinants of health outside the healthcare system, and random variation. Detecting quality differences on the basis of outcome measures usually takes a long time to observe,[17] and/or combining multiple outcomes into composite indicators.[19] Patient-reported outcomes may pick up more variation than standard outcomes,[20] but such measures remain relatively uncommon due to the effort required to collect them.

Casemix adjustment (also called 'risk adjustment') constitutes the most well-known challenge for outcomes-based quality measurement. Casemix differences can arise from patterns of patient referral and socioeconomic differences across local communities. The challenge of how to adjust for differences in casemix was noted as long ago as the mid-nineteenth century with the publication of league tables for hospital mortality in England. As one commentator wrote at the time: 'Any comparison which ignores the difference between the apple-cheeked farm-laborers who seek relief at Stoke Pogis (probably for rheumatism and sore legs), and the wizzened [sic], red-herring-like mechanics of Soho or Southwark, who come from a London Hospital, is fallacious.'[21]

Casemix adjustment has of course improved over the ensuing 150 years, but problems are still common.[22] For instance, multiple potential casemix adjustment models may exist for the same condition, and they may produce very different performance results.[23] Assumptions and choices in methodology can also generate controversy when it comes to interpreting trends in risk-adjusted outcomes, as with a prominent US programme focused on hospital readmissions.[24,25]

One general problem involves the distinction between comorbid conditions and illness severity. Consider again the example of patients hospitalised with acute myocardial infarction (Box 1). Adjusting for casemix in this context means adjusting for prognosis – expected clinical outcomes – at the moment of patient arrival. That prognosis will reflect the severity of the heart attack itself (e.g. how much heart muscle has infarcted), but it will also depend on comorbid conditions (e.g. diabetes, past strokes, chronic kidney disease). Although illness severity and comorbid conditions both impact prognosis, comorbid conditions are easier to measure using diagnostic codes generated by current or past encounters with the healthcare system (i.e. 'administrative data'). But such easily accessed diagnostic information does not help capture the severity of the acute heart attack. A hospital caring for patients with many comorbid conditions will look like it has a casemix with a high risk for death even if many of the heart attacks are in fact mild. Meanwhile, a hospital caring for patients who arrive in shock due to depressed cardiac function but have no obvious comorbid conditions will look like it cares for low-risk patients. Interestingly, misleading performance measurement can sometimes occur even with perfect risk adjustment; the problem arises when hospitals have different proportions of high-risk patients.[26]

There is also the special problem of adjusting for socioeconomic status. Socioeconomic factors – the social determinants of health – increase risks for poor outcomes in ways beyond the direct control of the health system. For instance, hospitals serving economically disadvantaged communities may more often encounter patients who first present for medical attention at more advanced stages of illness. Quality-related challenges can stem from various sources, including systemic issues such as chronic underfunding alongside broader institutional factors. Adjusting for socioeconomic factors may prevent the identification of critical quality issues. This remains a complex issue; there are numerous examples of national performance measurement programmes inadvertently penalising hospitals whose mission focuses on helping marginalised patient populations.[27-30]

3 Measurement Approaches in Action

There are a multitude of data sources and approaches available for assessing quality, each with its unique strengths and limitations (Table 2). The efficacy of any approach depends on several crucial factors, including its intended purpose, the intended audience, the resources allocated for implementation, and the potential consequences of inaccuracies. These considerations encompass a range of elements, such as specific objectives, target stakeholders, resource allocation for measurement initiatives, and the implications of flawed assessments. A comprehensive assessment of measurement approaches requires a multifaceted perspective, recognising the dynamic interplay of the factors that shape utility and effectiveness.

Table 2 Advantages and disadvantages of data sources and measurement approaches for healthcare improvement

Categories of measurement	Description	Examples (country)	Advantages	Disadvantages
Administrative data	Diagnostic codes associated with hospital admission or ambulatory attendances captured for administrative purposes.	Hospital Episode Statistics (HES) database (United Kingdom). [48,49] National hospital mortality surveillance system (United Kingdom). [50] Medicare claims (United States). [29]	May be inexpensive (since the data are already collected). Available for multiple (usually all) providers of healthcare in a given region or country.	Accuracy/data quality issues – errors may balance out for big picture studies, but not for single institutions. [51] Lacking clinically relevant detail (e.g. for adequate casemix adjustment or legitimate contraindications for processes of care).
Data warehouse	Multiple data sources in a healthcare system integrated and linked in one comprehensive database (e.g. electronic medical record linked to	Incidence and trends of central line associated pneumothorax using radiograph report text search versus	Allows characterisation of problems and care patterns which no single database could have done adequately on its own.	Substantial investments of money and personnel to develop and maintain. Need for robust governance model and rules for

Table 2 (cont.)

Categories of measurement	Description	Examples (country)	Advantages	Disadvantages
	daily patient census, staffing assignments, supply chain, and accounting data).[52,53]	administrative database codes (Canada).[51] Combining spatial and temporal data for patients' journeys with data from electronic health records (EHR) to identify source of an infectious outbreak (United States).[54]	Large case numbers enhance power in evaluating rare and complex conditions and operations.	managing requests for data access.
Patient registries and national clinical audits	Used for a broad range of purposes in healthcare serving as an organised system for the collection, storage, retrieval, analysis, and dissemination of information on patients who have a particular	Sentinel Stroke National Audit Programme (United Kingdom). National Emergency Laparotomy Audit (United Kingdom). American College of Surgeons National Surgical Quality	Data can help identify areas where hospitals may be underperforming. Provides insight into clinical performance improvement interventions.	Interpreting data correctly requires analytic methodology geared to address the potential sources of bias that challenge observational studies and also requires checks of internal validity.

	disease, condition, or exposure.[55]	Improvement Program (ACS NSQIP) (United States).[56,57] Cystic Fibrosis Foundation Patient Registry (United States).[58] Quality registries for inflammatory bowel disease in adults and children (Sweden, Italy).[59,60]	Provides hospital-specific and nationwide trends and health outcomes.	Many factors may compromise data quality, such as vague specification of variables, poorly designed abstraction tools, and poor or missing recording of data in the chart. Implicit reviews may be biased by abstractors' experience, consistency,
Chart review	The time required to ascertain key elements and outcomes of care from unstructured text in medical records has largely limited chart review to research studies looking for signals of improvement over time.[61,62] Deployment of artificial	I-PASS handoff programme (United States, Canada).[65] Trigger tools to detect adverse events/harm (Canada, United States).[66,67] Evaluation of the Health Foundation's Safer Patients Initiative (SPI) (United Kingdom).[40]	Has the clinical detail to support judgements about the preventability of undesirable outcomes or the appropriateness of care.	

Table 2 (cont.)

Categories of measurement	Description	Examples (country)	Advantages	Disadvantages
	intelligence tools in electronic medical records may make this approach more practical for measuring the impact of improvement efforts.[63,64]	Reviews of avoidable hospital deaths (United Kingdom).[68]		attention to detail, and harshness of judgement. Explicit reviews may lack sensitivity. Time-consuming and costly.
Qualitative methods	Qualitative methods are used in research approaches that aim to understand the meanings people attach to their experiences of the social world, study people in their day-to-day settings, and use different methods of data collection (e.g. interviews, observation,	Focus groups and individual interviews (Australia).[70] Ethnography and structured observation (United Kingdom).[71] Documentary analysis.	Provides a deeper and contextualised understanding of different aspects of an improvement intervention, ranging from understanding the problem, designing an intervention, understanding how the intervention was implemented in practice, and examining the	Rigorous use of qualitative methods requires expertise to ensure their use aligns with a chosen methodological approach and relevant quality criteria.[72] Interviews, focus groups, and observations are time-consuming.

	Description	Examples	Strengths	Limitations
	focus groups, documentary analysis).[69]		impacts of the intervention. Allows for an understanding of the perceptions and experiences of key and/or range of stakeholders in the improvement process.	
Patient surveys	Measuring patient experience is key to understanding many quality issues; it recognises them as experts in their own care journeys and experiences. Surveys capture data through single or multiple questions at the time of the care experience or days/weeks after the visit	Net promoter scores/families and friends test (United Kingdom).[73] Hospital Consumer Assessment of Healthcare Providers and Systems (HCAHPS) (United States).[74,75]	Flexible tool that allows for different methods of gathering patients' feedback. Imposes little extra work on care teams/practices. A source of extensive patient feedback. Increases the emphasis placed on patient experience. Offers a simple approach to driving cultural change	Collecting and managing such large amounts of data is complex. Requires substantial investments of time and other limited resources to collect, collate, and report responses. Local sites are often focused solely on attaining adequate response rates and establishing the proportion of patients

Table 2 (cont.)

Categories of measurement	Description	Examples (country)	Advantages	Disadvantages
	via telephone, email, mail, in person, etc.		or improving quality of care.	who would or would not recommend them, rather than enabling a comparative measure of performance. Metrics may lack credibility or have little value for informing improvement efforts.
Publicly available patient feedback	Comments from patients about their experiences with care available on social media platforms and publicly available websites.	Aggregated patient feedback from NHS Choices, Care Opinion, Facebook, and X (Twitter) to develop collective judgement scores for acute hospitals and trusts in order to inform decisions about which organisations	Rich unstructured data (as opposed to structured patient surveys). May be inexpensive to collect (where the data are already collected); may be more expensive to analyse. Available for multiple (usually all) providers	Accuracy/data quality issues – errors may balance out for big picture studies, but not for single institutions.[51] Lacking clinically relevant detail (e.g. for adequate casemix adjustment or legitimate

might be prioritised for further oversight by regulators such as the Care Quality Commission in England (United Kingdom).[76]

of healthcare in a given region or country.

contraindications for processes of care).

3.1 The Importance of Using Multiple Data Sources

Measurement that aims to understand the nature and scope of quality problems, as well as their contributing factors, benefits from the use of multiple data sources. A study from the patient safety literature vividly illustrates this point.[31] The authors liken the challenge of characterising safety problems with the Indian proverb involving six blind men, each touching a different part of an elephant: a tusk, trunk, ear, body, leg, or tail. Each blind man assumes they are touching a different object based on the part of the elephant they touch: a spear, snake, fan, wall, tree, or rope. Similarly, different perspectives on safety problems emerge depending on whether one uses incident reporting, record review, patient complaints, or executive walk rounds.[32] In this patient safety study, clinical judgement accounted for 25% of malpractice claims but only 1% of incident reports (primarily involving falls and issues relating to patient identification). Executive walk rounds, however, highlighted problematic work environments ranging from broken sinks to dysfunctional information systems. For these reasons, the authors recommend using at least three of the various methods available for identifying and characterising patient safety problems.[31]

Qualitative evaluations of improvement interventions also benefit from using multiple data sources, which may include not only interviews (e.g. with patients and staff) but also a review of organisational documents associated with developing and sustaining the initiative, and directly observing the clinical or improvement processes of interest (for example, using ethnographic methods).[33–37] Qualitative data such as these, alone or in combination, can provide insights into how improvement interventions are experienced by patients and clinicians. They can also identify ways in which the interventions can be optimised and any barriers to change. Qualitative investigations may also provide explanations for why an intervention did or did not achieve its goals.[38,39]

It's not surprising that using different types of data provides a fuller picture of quality given the multidimensional and complex nature of healthcare. That said, the benefits offered by a 'full picture' of measures must be balanced against the risk of measurement burden (see Section 3.3).[40–42] In some circumstances, using a wide range of measures and data sources may become too onerous and could even adversely impact the quality of care delivered by taking up too much personnel time, energy, and resources.[43]

3.2 Creating a Family of Measures

So far, we have covered the use of multiple data sources for both qualitative and quantitative characterisations of quality problems. When it comes to evaluating improvement interventions, the key concept is having a 'family of measures' regardless of the types of data involved. We want this family to include measures that allow us to answer three key questions:

- Was it implemented successfully?
- Did the intervention succeed in achieving its intended aim?
- Did the intervention create any new problems?

Answering these questions requires fidelity measures (capturing how often patients received the intervention in the intended manner), measures of success (defined by the desired improvements), and balancing measures (to capture any potential unintended consequences). For instance, in evaluating the introduction of a computerised clinical decision support system[44] to reduce prescriptions for unnecessary antibiotics, the success measures will include measures of antibiotic use (maybe total prescriptions and/or average number of days of antibiotics per patient). To assess fidelity, we might capture the degree to which clinicians simply dismissed the computer alert. A balancing measure might include the duration of patient visits to see if appointments are taking longer because of the need for clinicians to explain the basis for not prescribing the antibiotics that patients expect. Patient dissatisfaction over not receiving antibiotics might be another balancing measure.

3.3 Avoiding Measurement Burden

Improvement interventions typically use multiple measures. However, it's crucial to also consider the potential impact and burden on patients and clinicians affected by the intervention. Teams may face challenges in developing a robust measurement plan, defining measures clearly, and conducting reliable data collection and analysis.[45] They often choose unreliable or inappropriate measures, including locally developed ones, which may not align with validated measures needed for credible evidence.[45] Despite training, many teams lack the necessary skills for data collection and analysis.[45]

A common recommendation in relation to improvement work is to collect just enough data, avoiding the tendency (common in clinical research) to collect data just in case – i.e. in case the additional data might prove useful or interesting to analyse for purposes other than the main research question. When evaluating a healthcare improvement intervention, it's also not appropriate to make data collection difficult for the patients receiving care or the clinicians delivering it. There should be just enough data collected to ensure adequate evaluation of the intervention's intended and potential unintended consequences. Collecting additional data just in case they might prove interesting or inform some secondary questions will usually spell disaster.

Carefully considering the necessity of data collection is imperative. Suppose, for example, that a clinic wants to carry out an intervention aiming to improve medication adherence and avoid medication errors by encouraging patients to communicate more about their medicines. While it might seem tempting to survey patients and/or clinicians before and after the intervention to gauge changes in attitudes and assess the intervention's effectiveness, low response rates and the time burdens imposed on patients and clinicians could prevent successful implementation.

Although there's no recipe for how best to achieve adequate assessment using a family of measures while avoiding measurement burden, reflecting on the 'theory' of the intervention[46,47] and how it will achieve the intended improvement can help. We discuss this in the following section.

3.4 Using Theory to Inform Measurement Choices

As we have seen, a family of measures is usually needed to adequately assess the intended and unintended consequences of any improvement intervention. However, the process of data collection can pose challenges, potentially burdening patients or care providers. While no simple recipe exists for striking the optimal balance between these competing concerns, clearly articulating a plausible theory for how an intervention is expected to achieve its objectives can guide our decision-making.[46,47] In fact, a recent commentary outlines 'five golden rules' for measurement for improvement, the first of which advises explaining a plausible theory for how a proposed change will achieve the desired improvement.[77]

To illustrate the ways in which the theory for an intervention can inform measurement choices, we can consider a patient-empowerment intervention to improve clinicians' adherence to hand hygiene.[78] The intervention consists of telling patients that they should feel empowered to ask whether a clinician has washed their hands before an examination. This intervention may at first seem like it works as a kind of reminder. But it is not a reminder in the usual sense. Rather it is a 'sticky reminder' – one that is not expected to be delivered often to any given clinician. But, when it is delivered, the theory of the intervention is that they will remember for a long time. Why? Because most health professionals will feel some shame over a patient pointing out such a basic oversight. So, the theory for this 'sticky reminder' is that it will have an impact far beyond any single delivery – that the embarrassing memory of being caught neglecting basic hygiene will lead to improved compliance in the future.

This is a plausible theory; one can reasonably expect that the intervention could achieve its goal improving hand hygiene. But, clearly explaining that the intervention's success depends on patients delivering a mild form of professional embarrassment suggests two important implementation issues to address: patients may not feel comfortable challenging/embarrassing clinicians, and clinicians may sometimes react negatively.[79] The implementation plan will need to address these issues. The family of measures (see Section 3.2) will also need to include balancing measures that assess the degree to which patients ever encountered negative reactions from clinicians or perceived that their speaking up adversely affected their care.

Thinking through the theory of an intervention also helps develop another element in the family of measures, namely capturing fidelity or implementation success. In order for the hand hygiene intervention to have any hope of working, patients first need to be aware of the new policy encouraging them to feel comfortable speaking up when they think a clinician entering their hospital room has not used one of the nearby hand hygiene dispensers or washed their hands at a sink in the room. An improvement team implementing this intervention might initially choose to encourage awareness among patients using posters announcing this patient empowerment campaign, placed strategically in locations throughout the hospital. The chance that this would reach enough patients seems small. But the improvement team is hesitant to take the step of asking nurses and/or physicians to tell patients about this policy as part of their workflow for every new patient encounter. To add to the chance that the poster campaign will work, clinicians are encouraged to wear lapel badges depicting two hands surrounded by soap bubbles and delivering the line 'Ask me if I have washed my hands!' The team reasons that this step will help increase awareness of the campaign not only among patients but also among clinicians. To assess the degree to which these steps have achieved adequate awareness, the improvement team decides to check in with five patients per ward every week to ask if they are aware of the new policy and if they have ever asked a clinician if they have washed their hands. While on any given hospital unit performing this audit, the member of the improvement team will also make note of the rough proportion of clinicians wearing one of the intervention buttons.

Each of these steps may seem 'obvious'. But they are easy to overlook unless we deliberately think through how a given intervention is expected to work. By thinking through the theory for an intervention it will usually become clear what is needed to measure successful implementation and possible negative consequences of the intervention. The theory for an intervention also helps with another key aspect of measurement – suggesting a plausible timeline for success.[77] Most interventions do not work like light switches that, once switched on, immediately produce the desired change. Computer alerts and other forms of decision support for clinicians[44] represent a rare case of improvement 'light switches': whatever effect the alert will have can be expected to occur as soon as the hospital informatics team turns it on. But most interventions depend on a number of steps successfully occurring in order for the desired change to have a reasonable chance of taking place. In the hand hygiene example, these steps included developing a strategy for making patients aware that they should feel comfortable asking clinicians if they have washed their hands, as well as preparing clinicians so that they do not react negatively due to being caught off guard.

Other interventions, such as those depending on substantial changes of attitudes among clinicians and/or managers, could take months or even years for key steps to take hold. For instance, the mechanisms of action for central line bundles and the surgical checklist probably depend on changes to attitudes and behaviours beyond those suggested just by the technical elements on these checklists.[80] Without such changes, clinicians will treat key items on the checklist, such as taking time out before the procedure to verify the correct patient and procedure, like a tick box exercise, which will achieve little.[81,82] Identifying the need for widespread changes in attitude makes it clear that this intervention could take months or years to take hold. The family of measures will also need to include elements that assess the degree to which these necessary changes in attitude are occurring.

4 Validity Considerations in Measurement

4.1 Types of Validity

The different types of validity – face, content, construct, criterion, and convergent (Box 2) – and associated terminology can be confusing. Although these considerations can seem like they would apply only to research studies, the different forms of validity also apply to improvement efforts. For instance, does the measure make conceptual sense in terms of capturing the quality problem of interest (face validity)? Does the measure adequately capture all relevant dimensions of the target problem (content validity)? And do the results of the measure in practice reflect the concept of interest – or something else? Even 'minimum bias', which sounds very research oriented, amounts to addressing the problem that performance at one hospital can look much better than elsewhere just because its patients are not at particularly high risk of bad outcomes.

Suppose an independent agency contacts patients shortly after they have left hospital and asks the single survey question: 'Were you satisfied with the care you received in the hospital?' Put aside for the moment the question of whether the answer is a simple yes/no or a five-point Likert scale that allows for a more graded response. For our purposes, just consider if asking patients a question about their satisfaction seems reasonable as a measure of patient satisfaction.

Box 2 Types of Validity and Key Concepts to Consider[83,84]

- **Face validity**

  The degree to which a measure makes sense in principle as capturing the quality problem it intends to describe. Face validity is similar to content validity but is more subjective.

- **Content validity**

  The conceptual soundness of a measure, or the extent to which a measure's content captures all aspects of the concept of interest.

- **Construct validity**

  Establishes whether the measure empirically captures the theoretical concept envisioned.

- **Criterion validity**

  The degree of correlation or agreement of the measure with an independent criterion or gold standard (concurrent validity) or against a future standard (predictive validity).

- **Convergent validity**

  The degree to which a given measure agrees with related measures (and disagrees with or diverges from unrelated measures).

- **Precision**

  Is there a substantial amount of provider-level or community-level variation not attributable to random variation?

- **Minimum bias**

  Is there either little effect from variations in casemix, or is it possible to apply risk adjustment and statistical methods to minimise such bias?

- **Fosters real improvement**

  Is the indicator insulated from perverse incentives for providers to improve their reported performance by avoiding difficult or complex cases, or by other responses that do not improve quality of care? For instance, more thorough documentation of chronic medical problems will make patients seem sicker and increase their 'expected mortality'. A hospital will then appear to have lowered their hospital standardised mortality (the ratio of actual to expected deaths) even if no reduction in actual deaths has occurred.

This is not a trick question. On the face of it, it seems reasonable enough, so measuring the percentage of patients answering such a question positively has face validity. Interviewing patients or analysing their comments on social media[76,85] could also produce measures of patient satisfaction with face validity. But for each such measure, we need to recognise that patient satisfaction may depend on distinct elements of care – clarity of communication, attentiveness of staff, cleanliness of the hospital room, and so on.

A measure with face validity and conceptually sound content validity still needs to be assessed to see the degree to which it captures the concept of interest in practice; this is referred to as its construct validity. The concept of interest here is patient satisfaction itself – the degree to which patients are satisfied with the care they received in the hospital. However, patient satisfaction can be influenced by various elements of care, including communication clarity, staff attentiveness, and hospital cleanliness. Even though these measures may seem conceptually sound and have face validity, we must evaluate their construct validity – how well they accurately capture the concept of interest in real-world practice. A patient might report high overall satisfaction despite encountering failings in specific aspects of care, particularly if their treatment outcomes were successful. This highlights the possibility that measures of patient satisfaction may not fully encompass all relevant aspects of the target concept. When the measures are imperfect, it makes sense to consider convergent validity – whether different tools or tests that are supposed to measure the same thing actually do so consistently. For instance, hospital mortality, readmissions rates, and patient volumes are all imperfect measures. Showing agreement with each other could be seen as validating them to some extent. A national study of surgical patients examined 30-day readmission rates after hospitalisation for six types of major surgery. Hospitals in the highest quartile for surgical volume (a known structural measure of quality[9-11,86]) had a significantly lower readmission rate than hospitals in the lowest quartile. Similarly, hospitals with the lowest mortality rates had significantly lower readmission rates than hospitals with the highest mortality rates.[87] In this case, there are also conceptual reasons to support this convergent validity. Surgical readmissions commonly involve post-operative complications occurring shortly after discharge,[88] and prevention strategies exist for many of these complications (e.g. surgical site infections).

4.2 Application of Validity Concepts across Measures

Table 3 comments on the content validity and construct validity for three quality measures where high-quality primary care can reduce the risk of emergency hospitalisations:

Table 3 Content and Construct Validity for Case Example Quality Measures

Example measure	Target quality problem and rationale	Content validity	Construct validity
Hip fracture surgery in patients admitted to hospital with a principal diagnosis other than hip fracture.*	Patients are usually not admitted to hospital with a plan to undergo a major operation or medical treatment and repair a fractured hip. Therefore, any hospitalisation where this occurred must reflect an admission complicated by an in-hospital fall resulting in hip fracture.	While this measure does not capture all fall-related injuries, it does make conceptual sense that any cases flagged by this indicator involved hip fractures from falls that occurred in hospital. *Content validity thus seems present for this measure.*	Medical record review confirms that this measure captures its intended target for surgical patients. For medical patients, though, it often turns out that the patient was admitted with a hip fracture after all. [92]
Hospital standardised mortality ratio (HSMR): the ratio of observed mortality at a given hospital to the	Deficiencies in hospital care contributing to an increased risk of death should be detectable by observing more deaths at a given	Generating an expected mortality represents a deceptively complex scientific task. [94,95] Even with perfect casemix adjustment, hospitals with	More careful coding of patient risk factors will lower the HSMR by increasing the denominator (expected deaths) even if the numerator

Table 3 (cont.)

Example measure	Target quality problem and rationale	Content validity	Construct validity
mortality expected based on the hospital's casemix.	hospital than would be expected from its patient population – including its demographic factors (e.g. age, gender) and comorbid conditions.	different proportions of high-risk patients will look like they differ in quality even when they do not.[26] Finally, most in-hospital deaths do not result from deficient care.[68,96] On the other hand, most deficient care does not produce death. *Content validity thus seems questionable.*	(observed deaths) remains unchanged. The choice of measurement instrument – the particular casemix adjustment tool and set of inclusion and exclusion criteria for case selection – has substantial impact on the results.[23] *Construct validity thus seems questionable*
Hospital admissions for ambulatory care sensitive conditions (ACSCs).[97]	There are medical conditions for which timely and effective outpatient care can help to reduce the risks of hospitalisation by either preventing deterioration (e.g. optimal asthma or	The original study proposing ACSCs showed the 'impact of socioeconomic differences on rates of hospitalisation' and concluded that 'the lack of timely and effective outpatient care may lead to	Many studies highlight the degree to which socio-economic factors, such as neighbourhood deprivation and education levels, have substantial impacts on

diabetes management to avoid exacerbations requiring hospitalisation) or prompting outpatient treatment of cellulitis or gastroenteritis before they become severe enough to require hospitalisation.

higher hospitalisation rates in low-income areas'.[98] *Thus, ACSCs have limited content validity as a measure of ambulatory care quality.* They probably say more about deprivation and the lack of timely access to any ambulatory care rather than the quality of ambulatory care delivered by the clinics in a hospital's catchment area.

variation in ACSCs across hospitals.[99-102]

---

* This example indicator represents a simplified version of *PSI 08 In Hospital Fall with Hip Fracture Rate*, one of the Patient Safety Indicators produced by the US Agency for Healthcare Research and Quality.[103]

- Injurious inpatient falls (hip fracture surgery in patients admitted to hospital for another reason)
- Hospital standardised mortality ratios (HSMR)
- Hospital admissions for ambulatory care sensitive conditions (ACSCs – outpatient conditions such as diabetes, asthma, and congestive heart failure, among others).

(Table 3 does not comment on face validity because its subjective nature makes it the weakest form of validity.)

The measure intended to capture in-hospital fractures makes sense conceptually (content validity) and is likely to measure what it intends to measure (construct validity) in surgical patients. But for medical patients, a substantial number of cases identified by this measure involve patients who were admitted to the hospital with a pre-existing hip fracture, rather than fractures occurring during their hospital stay due to falls. The other two measures – the HSMR and ACSCs – have limited or questionable face validity, and both end up having measurement problems that undermine their construct validity.

ACSCs aim to measure the quality of ambulatory (outpatient) care using widely available administrative data associated with hospital admissions – specifically, admissions for conditions where better care might have avoided the need for hospitalisation. They are an example of a measure whose widespread use likely reflects its availability rather than its conceptual soundness or performance in practice. The data necessary to assess the quality of ambulatory care directly are often not easily available across all ambulatory practices in a given region. The measure reflects the ease of obtaining hospital episode statistics, such as emergency department visits and hospital admissions with basic diagnostic codes (e.g. 'asthma' or 'diabetes'). It is much harder to directly assess the quality of ambulatory care a patient has received for diabetes than it is to measure simply that they visited the emergency department or were admitted to hospital for a diagnosis that possibly involved their diabetes.

Despite the use of ACSCs to assess ambulatory care quality, it's important to recognise that ambulatory care may not fully address all essential elements of established healthcare practices.[89,90] This understanding is crucial, especially given that efforts to improve care for exactly the type of chronic conditions targeted by ACSCs, such as diabetes, often yield only modest improvements.[91]

The Patient Safety Indicators (PSIs) developed by the US Agency for Healthcare Research Quality are widely used measures, primarily due to the ease of accessing necessary administrative data, rather than their validity. One of these indicators, represented by the first measure in Table 3 – hip fracture surgery in patients admitted to hospital with a principal diagnosis other than hip fracture – represents a simplified version of one of these indicators. The intent of this indicator lies in detecting the patient safety problem of inpatient falls resulting in an injury. The indicator is meant to detect patients who fell while in hospital and broke their hip (i.e. the safety problem of inpatient falls resulting in serious injury, one of the most common of which is a broken hip). The idea makes conceptual sense: look for patients who were admitted for anything other than hip surgery and, if they also underwent hip surgery while in hospital, it probably reflects an inpatient fall resulting in a broken hip. This makes sense because no one is admitted to hospital to have their gallbladder removed (or undergo heart surgery or whatever the case may be) and undergo hip surgery during the same admission. But, for medical patients, it's not uncommon for, say, an elderly patient to have collapsed (e.g. they fainted from low blood pressure caused by early sepsis) and broken their hip in the process. So, when these patients admitted for medical conditions undergo hip surgery, they are flagged as cases of broken hips due to inpatient falls (the target safety problem) even though the fall happened prior to the admission. This patient safety indicator – undergoing hip surgery during hospitalisations for any principal diagnosis not involving the hip – has content validity and has construct validity for surgical patients but performs very poorly for medical patients[92]. In fact, a systematic review of literature found that only one PSI (accidental puncture and laceration during a surgical procedure) had a true positive rate of at least 80%.[93] (The 'true positive rate' refers to the proportion of cases correctly identified as having the complication of interest by the indicator.) For all the other indicators, medical record review confirmed the complication of interest for fewer than 80% of cases flagged by the indicator.

4.3 Measurement Specification and Operationalisation

Even a valid measure can run into problems when it has not been well-specified. Consider a team aiming to improve medication safety using a care bundle related to medication reconciliation (accurately listing a person's current medicines) and review. The quality problem they want to address is unintended discrepancies between medications patients receive in hospital compared with what they have been taking at home. Hospital-based physicians often make deliberate changes to these medicines based on issues related to the acute illness. But they can also inadvertently make changes because they don't have easy access to patients' complete pre-admission medication lists. The improvement team decides to make its main measure of success the '[n]umber of patients who have their medicines 100% correct 24 hours into their hospital stay'. This measure has validity given the aims of the improvement initiative, but will serve little purpose without specifying how staff should establish correctness.[45] An operational definition is needed that includes the specific sources of information those conducting the measurement should consult and other key steps to determine the correct medicine list for a given patient.

Another example comes from a study of improvement teams engaged in a national initiative to reduce central venous catheter bloodstream infections (CVC-BSI).[104] The main measure consisted of the monthly CVC-BSI rate, defined as the monthly number of bloodstream infections per 1,000 CVC patient days. Calculating this infection rate requires dividing the number of bloodstream infections (the numerator) by the number of CVC patient days (the denominator) and multiplying by 1,000. Even at this stage, there is already some complexity involving the denominator, as it requires counting all patients with CVCs and counting how many CVCs each patient had. This counting requires some standardisation, such as specifying a time of day for when it should happen. There also needs to be an operational protocol that provides guidance for what to do if a patient is not available at the time designated for counting CVCs (e.g. because the patient is undergoing a procedure).

Determining the numerator for the CVC-BSI rate also requires a protocol providing clear guidance on identifying relevant infections.[104] There again needs to be a specified time of day for when this counting should occur. And, similar to the above medication example, there needs to be a protocol specifying the steps to be taken to identify relevant data elements from clinical notes and microbiological test results. There also needs to be a clear definition of what constitutes an infection in terms of the various possible combinations of these data elements. Some patients may have blood culture results indicating a bacteria which can cause CVC-BSIs, but the clinical team may have determined in a given case that it was a 'contaminant' (i.e. skin bacteria that contaminated the needle used to collect the blood sample). On the other hand, there are times when doctors will treat a patient for a suspected CVC-BSI even if the blood culture doesn't show a positive result. In this case, even with acceptable combinations of relevant data elements clearly specified, some cases may remain ambiguous, so the protocol would need to indicate when to involve others to judge a given potential CVC-BSI.

Measures involving any judgement of delay or elapsed time will also require clear specification. For instance, in Box 1 we mentioned door-to-balloon and door-to-needle times, common process of care measures for the quality of care delivered to patients with acute myocardial infarction and stroke. These measures need clear specification of details such as when the 'clock starts ticking'. For door-to-balloon time, consensus guidelines indicate that the clock starts ticking the moment the patient arrives at the hospital (the 'door' time). A protocol for measurement needs to clearly specify the appropriate data sources for establishing this door time. It also needs to include clear guidance on how to handle various situations. For instance, if a patient first presents to a hospital that is not equipped to perform percutaneous coronary intervention (PCI) and then is transferred to a PCI-capable facility, the initial door time could be at the first hospital, or the arrival time at the second hospital. Practices may vary, and clear guidelines are essential to ensure consistency in measurement. In cases where emergency medical services notify the receiving hospital while on the way there, the protocol needs to specify if the door time should in fact consist of this notification time instead of physical arrival at the hospital. Similar considerations give rise to the need for clear specification of details related to the 'balloon' time, the key step in the PCI procedure.

4.4 Sampling Considerations

Improvement teams also need to consider sampling in their improvement work, particularly how sampling strategies in improvement differ from those used in research. A frequent pitfall in healthcare improvement is collecting too much data when local gaps in care can be demonstrated with very small sample sizes.[105] In evaluative clinical trials, the goal is to detect statistically significant differences among groups, with high precision. By contrast, healthcare improvement work often aims to determine if local performance is meeting a specific standard. When performance is poor, small samples may be enough to show that local care is falling short of an expected standard. For instance, suppose current practice guidelines recommend that 80% of patients receive some process of care, and an audit of 12 eligible patients shows this guideline is being met just 50% of the time. Even with this small sample size, the 95% confidence interval for this point estimate of 6 out of 12 does not include the desired performance of 80%.[105]

As with any sampling, it is essential to consider representativeness and the degree to which observations include factors that may contribute to variation, such as clinical variables (e.g. illness severity, comorbid conditions), day of week, time of day, ethnic diversity, and so on. But data quality is especially important when using small samples to ensure validity of results and to make reasonable assumptions about local system performance. Important considerations for achieving high data quality and integrity are outlined in Box 3.

Box 3 Key Steps to Consider When Using Small Samples in Improvement[105]

1. **Define the eligible sample**
   While random samples are ideal, they are usually impractical for most improvement projects. For feasibility of recruitment, consider enrolling consecutive eligible patients or using convenience samples.

2. **Establish exclusion criteria**
   Be clear and explicit about the basis on which you would exclude those patients for whom the audit or improvement efforts do not apply.

3. **State your study period**
   State clearly the start and end times for the audit/improvement cycle.

4. **Keep a reject log**
   Keep track of patients who were excluded and the reasons for doing so.

5. **Make data collection complete**
   Ensuring completeness of data collection is of paramount importance, as sometimes the reason for missing/incomplete data relates to the target quality problem.

5 Concepts and Problems Unique to Measurement for Healthcare Improvement

In the previous section, we covered issues that are likely to arise in the context of measurement in any discipline. But when measurement occurs in the context of assessing healthcare quality – especially in the context of efforts to improve healthcare quality – then distinct problems can arise. No framework is available for organising these problems, nor is there necessarily even agreement on what to call them. Those engaged in improvement efforts will encounter them, so we offer the following descriptions.

5.1 Surveillance Bias

Surveillance bias, also known as detection or ascertainment bias, occurs when one group of subjects is followed up more closely than others – for example, those who undergo a medical treatment or test.[106,107] Surveillance bias can arise whenever an outcome depends on clinical (or institutional) behaviours. For example, in a clinical trial with venous thromboembolism (VTE – a blood clot that forms in a vein which partially or completely obstructs blood flow) as an outcome, the trial protocol will systematically determine the outcome of interest in all patients, but, as the study described in Box 4 shows, when evaluating the quality of care related to VTE, the outcome of interest may reflect how carefully clinicians test for it.

Surveillance bias may occur consciously, but it may also reflect other initiatives occurring at the same time. For instance, reducing catheter-related urinary tract infection (CAUTI) has become a common target of hospital improvement efforts, and the checklist of actions to prevent CAUTI include elements that should reduce UTI.[109] But hospitals have also sought to reduce unnecessary testing, including the so-called pan culture – i.e. the ordering of blood and urine cultures any time a patient's clinical status worsens, even if there is no real suspicion of sepsis or a UTI.[110] The definition of CAUTI requires a positive urine culture. Thus, if the rate of obtaining urine cultures falls due to these (appropriate) stewardship efforts, then rates of CAUTI will also decrease regardless of any impact of the preventive CAUTI actions. One multifaceted improvement effort targeting the reduction of CAUTIs in intensive care units (ICUs) involved aligning routine culturing practices with guidelines for evaluating fever in critically ill patients, leading to a notable decrease in CAUTI rates.[111] This example illustrates how changes in culturing practices, driven by

---

BOX 4 SURVEILLANCE BIAS OF THE VENOUS THROMBOEMBOLISM QUALITY MEASURE

Bilimoria et al.[108] examined whether surveillance bias influences the validity of reported VTE rates. They found that hospitals with higher rates of evidence-based VTE preventive action (i.e. hospitals that would score highly on this process-based measure of hospital quality) also had higher rates of actual VTE (i.e. they would score poorly on the outcome-based measure of quality).

The benefits of VTE preventive action in reducing VTE have been established in multiple randomised controlled trials. In this case, the unexpected lack of consistency between the process and outcome of interest turned out to reflect clinicians' behaviour in ordering tests. Clinicians in hospitals that delivered VTE preventive action more consistently also ordered the tests more often, paradoxically worsening their hospital's VTE quality measure performance.

The direction of effect for surveillance bias cannot necessarily be predicted on conceptual grounds. In this case, for example, one might reasonably have speculated that clinicians at a hospital with high rates of delivering VTE preventive action would think it less necessary to check for VTE, as the chance of it occurring ought to be lower.

initiatives targeting different aspects of patient care, can inadvertently impact the reported rates of CAUTIs.

To protect against surveillance bias, it's important to ask if the measure depends on the behaviours of clinicians or patients. The possibility of bias is usually obvious for patient-reported outcomes. For instance, an ambulatory clinic with a low number of patient complaints (compared with other clinics) may reflect high-quality, patient-centred care. But it could also reflect a patient population that does not feel comfortable speaking up about shortcomings in their care, or the clinic may not even have told patients how to make a complaint. So other means of obtaining information from patients also need to be considered, such as a formal survey or harnessing social media and looking for comments about the clinic in question.[112,113] In other words, for some types of surveillance bias additional data sources are needed for the same outcome.

This concept comes up again in Box 5, which demonstrates the need for multiple data sources rather than relying exclusively on voluntary incident reporting when measuring patient falls in hospital. But the VTE example discussed in Box 4 offers a different solution to the same problem: choose a different outcome. Among those factors that may give rise to in-hospital VTE, the main intervention within the control of clinicians (or the hospital as a whole) is appropriate preventive action. Rather than measure the occurrence of VTE, which depends in part on how carefully clinicians pursue the diagnosis of VTE, just measure the provision of appropriate preventive action. The relevant prescribing data are available in the medical record and are not subject to surveillance bias.

5.2 Interventions That by Their Nature Directly Affect or Change the Outcome

Some interventions, by their nature, change how we measure outcomes. For example, suppose one designs a computerised alert to reduce a particular medication error.[59] Before the alert has been implemented, you might carefully review records to identify all errors (the numerator) and total number of patients receiving the medication (the denominator). After the intervention, you might simply use how often the alert triggers as the total number of patients and the instances where clinicians didn't follow its recommendation as the number of errors. This difference in how we measure outcomes introduces errors that are difficult to adjust for in analysis. To mitigate this, an improvement team might run the computer alert in the background before the intervention starts, ensuring consistent measurement methods.

Another potential example of this problem can be seen in efforts to improve sepsis care. Sepsis is well-known to carry a high mortality rate – probably about 20% for hospitalised patients.[114] Improvement interventions for sepsis often encourage identification of subtler, less severe cases. But less severely ill patients are the ones more likely to be missed in the pre-intervention period, so the post-intervention mortality rate will have a denominator that includes patients who differ in their risk of death from those in the pre-intervention period. Clinical trials avoid this problem by having clear criteria for sepsis – and clinical trials on this topic tend to show that the types of protocols championed for sepsis improvement efforts do not improve outcomes,[115] further calling into question the results of improvement interventions that have apparently reduced sepsis mortality.

When this problem of an intervention changing the outcome of interest arises, there is no easy way to avoid it, beyond recognising it and resisting the temptation to exploit it. So it is better to report the degree to which an improvement intervention has increased the proportion of patients receiving care that follows the guidelines for sepsis and not trumpet that the intervention has also achieved substantial reductions in mortality from sepsis. To pursue the latter claim, it would be necessary to apply validated prognostic tools for categorising patients' risk of death. Such methods are routinely applied in clinical research on critically ill patients, but they remain uncommon in quality improvement efforts.

5.3 Need for Multiple Data Sources to Characterise Measure of Interest

In quality improvement interventions, identifying patients with specific conditions or complications often requires more effort than clinical research. This difference reflects the historic focus in medical records on clearly documenting diagnoses and treatments. For instance, a clinical researcher interested in acute myocardial infarctions (heart attacks) can fairly easily identify all such patients from laboratory data (involving blood levels of cardiac enzymes released from damaged heart muscle). They can also easily call up data on key medications delivered to patients who have been admitted with heart attacks. Patients admitted with a heart attack will almost always have this as their principal discharge diagnosis, so administrative data will provide a fairly easy way of identifying the patients of interest. A clinical researcher interested in heart attacks has multiple options, each of which works easily and well. By contrast, consider the person interested in a very common hospital-acquired complication – injurious falls. Some of these injuries will result in fractures, but many will not, so test results will give an incomplete picture. The discharge diagnoses for these patients commonly miss out mentioning this event. And, the voluntary incident reporting systems hospitals run are notoriously problematic in terms of under detecting the problems of interest.[116] Because of this, anyone interested in improvement in this context needs to employ a 'triangulation' approach, using multiple data sources such as incident reporting, chart review, and natural language searching of radiologic results to identify patients with the quality problem of injurious falls among hospitalised patients. An example of this approach is described in Box 5.

CAUTI is another common hospital-acquired condition where multiple data sources may be required to measure outcomes. Defining the outcome presents several challenges. Patients can have catheters inserted without an obvious (or always reliable) trace being left in a single part of the medical record, so the at-risk group (the denominator for the eventual CAUTI rate) requires multiple data sources or prospective surveillance as part of an infection control initiative. And while it is tempting to use the decision to treat (i.e. an order for antibiotics) as a basis for the numerator, not all positive urine cultures reflect true infections – yet clinicians may choose to treat them anyway. So determining the numerator of all CAUTIs requires more than one data source (e.g. chart review to identify the presence of factors deemed by expert consensus to indicate true cases of CAUTI).

5.4 Outcomes that Suffer from Incomplete Data Capture

Some outcomes, by their nature, suffer from incomplete data capture. This problem commonly occurs in relation to diagnostic errors, including diagnoses that were initially missed but later identified and diagnoses that were never identified or corrected. This latter group can potentially be identified for the minority of delayed diagnoses with high risks of near-term morbidity and mortality. Among patients assessed in emergency departments for dizziness, for example, a small percentage are discharged with missed posterior circulation strokes. Looking at subsequent healthcare visits within 30 days will identify some of these missed diagnoses.[120] But with most diagnostic errors, there is no easy way of addressing this problem. When clinicians do not consider a particular diagnosis likely, it will not be actively pursued, which means the medical record will contain no definitive test making clear that the patient did not have the diagnosis of interest. This amounts to a type of ascertainment or surveillance bias.

'Wrong-patient orders' in computerised physician order entry systems provide a clear example of an intrinsically incomplete outcome. Here, the event of interest is entering an order – for medication or an investigation – on the wrong patient. There are several possible causes – having more than one record open,

---

Box 5 Using Triangulation to Ascertain Fall Injuries in Acute Hospitals

Barker et al. used a triangulation approach to determine outcomes in their cluster randomised controlled trial (RCT) evaluating an intervention to reduce injurious falls in hospitals.[117] The 6-PACK programme included use of a nine-item fall risk tool and individualised use of one or more of the following six interventions:

- A fall alert sign (to alert staff to patients at high risk of falling)
- Supervision of patients in the bathroom
- Ensuring patients' walking aids were within reach
- A toileting regimen
- Use of a low-low bed
- Use of a bed/chair alarm.

The intervention was quite plausible and evidence-based, and it did show positive changes in fall prevention practice; however, no difference was seen in falls or fall injuries.

In contrast, Dykes et al.'s study focused solely on voluntary incident reporting to identify injurious falls, which reported a 34% reduction in such falls.[118] Despite similarities in the intervention elements between the two studies, Dykes' study lacked the use of multiple methods for determining the outcomes. Although the positive study used a non-randomised design, it was a stepped wedge trial involving 14 medical units within three academic medical centres in two cities – i.e. about as close to an RCT as one could hope as the units are in both treatment arms at different times. So rather than a study design problem, the positive result here more likely reflects the difference in outcome ascertainment, with the positive study using a single data source – a source known to say more about reporting behaviour and organisational culture than about the underlying event rate of interest.[119] Dykes' study relied solely on a single data source, which is recognised for its potential biases related to reporting behaviour and organisational culture rather than providing an accurate reflection of the true event rate of interest.

---

selecting the next patient on a patient roster list, or patients having similar names, for example. The measure that has emerged in evaluations of various potential interventions is 'retract-and-reorder':[121,122] investigators designed an electronic query to identify orders that were placed for a patient but retracted within a short time interval (e.g. 10 minutes) and then reordered shortly afterwards by the same clinician for a different patient. But this measure necessarily misses wrong patient orders that are not recognised so quickly or at all.

5.5 Engaging Stakeholders in Measure Development

Interventions are often implemented without thorough consideration of their efficacy or potential drawbacks. This oversight is highlighted by the tendency to prioritise rapid implementation over comprehensive analysis and measurement. In addition, the heterogeneity of quality targets – and the wide range of issues that can arise depending on the specifics of any given intervention and the context for its evaluation – makes it difficult to set out all the problems that might arise and to offer a comprehensive list of strategies for avoiding them. To address these challenges effectively, practitioners should consider the five golden rules for measurement:

- Understanding the theory of change
- Identifying fidelity/process measures
- Selecting appropriate measurement methods
- Considering lag time for outcomes
- Anticipating unintended consequences.[77]

By explicitly explaining mechanisms of effect and associated theories of change early in project development, practitioners can develop more effective interventions. This proactive approach ensures that interventions are not only deployed as intended but also evaluated comprehensively for their impact on patient care and safety.

We have provided, throughout the material above, some potential mitigation strategies for the problems discussed. But although it is not possible to list mitigation strategies for all potential measurement problems, a good general rule is always to involve stakeholders in co-creating the measures. For instance, ask clinicians subject to the measures of interest if they see them as capturing the underlying concepts of interest, if the measures will unfairly penalise certain clinicians or patient groups, and if the measures create perverse incentives or have obvious opportunities for manipulation. In many situations, it will be necessary to ask similar questions of patient representatives, while taking care to avoid tokenism.[123] In other words, make sure you obtain input from a representative range of patients.

6 Conclusion

For any given quality problem, no single measure or measurement method will provide the complete picture. The first step is to consider the primary purpose of the measurement – for instance, is the measurement primarily for accountability (e.g. public reporting) or for fostering and informing improvement interventions? But regardless of purpose, basic considerations include the degree to which a measure makes conceptual sense (face validity), captures the concept of interest (construct validity), and exhibits other forms of validity discussed in this Element. Other considerations include the degree to which variations in casemix, chance effects, and perverse incentives or gaming can affect the measures of interest. Improvement efforts also generate some unique measurement issues: for instance, organisations and places with more apparent quality problems could truly be delivering worse care; alternatively, they might be looking for and documenting such problems more comprehensively than their peers.

Evaluating improvement efforts usually requires a family of measures. For instance, an intervention for reducing fall-related injuries among hospitalised patients might need the following:

- Multiple data sources to identify injurious falls, including incident reports, chart notes, and radiology reports
- Fidelity measures capturing the degree to which patients received the various prevention strategies
- Balancing measures to look for unintended consequences (e.g. were physical or pharmacologic restraints used more often?).

But it is also important to avoid imposing overly demanding measurement on patients, clinicians, or organisations affected by the intervention. Don't collect measures just in case they might inform future research; instead, collect just enough data to support the evaluation. Clearly explaining a plausible theory for how the intervention is expected to achieve its intended results can also help inform choices about the amount and types of measurement to pursue. Finally, for any given measure, obtain input from the measurement subjects – clinicians or patients. This type of stakeholder engagement will often lead to improvement of the measure – but even when it doesn't, it will likely increase the acceptability of the eventual measurement results.

Considering the multifaceted nature of quality measurement, future research should focus on developing comprehensive approaches that address the diverse needs of stakeholders. This includes further exploration of methodologies for balancing measurement burden with the depth of evaluation required for improvement efforts. Additionally, research should delve into the impact of stakeholder engagement on measure refinement and implementation success. By prioritising stakeholder involvement and methodological innovation, future research can contribute to more effective quality improvement interventions.

7 Further Reading

- Batalden PB et al.[124] – defines quality improvement and the roadmap for improvement.
- Berwick DM et al.[125] – describes how to control variation in healthcare.
- Berwick DM et al.[126] – explains the connection between improvement, change, and learning as it relates to healthcare systems.
- Best M et al.[127] – outlines the origins of quality improvement.
- Langley GJ et al.[128] – describes the Model for Improvement, an integrated approach to process improvement that delivers quick and substantial results in quality and productivity in diverse settings.
- Provost LP et al.[129] – transforms raw data into concrete healthcare improvements.
- Etchells E et al.[105] – gives an overview on how small samples can make important contributions to improvement projects.

Contributors

Alene Toulany and Kaveh Shojania conceptualised the Element, drafted the initial outline, and wrote the Element collaboratively. Kaveh Shojania provided supervision, and both authors have approved the final version.

Conflicts of Interest

None.

Acknowledgements

We thank the peer reviewers for their insightful comments and recommendations to improve the Element.

Funding

This Element was funded by THIS Institute (The Healthcare Improvement Studies Institute, www.thisinstitute.cam.ac.uk). THIS Institute is strengthening the evidence base for improving the quality and safety of healthcare. THIS Institute is supported by a grant to the University of Cambridge from the Health Foundation – an independent charity committed to bringing about better health and healthcare for people in the United Kingdom.

About the Authors

Alene Toulany, MD MSc FRCPC, is an Adolescent Medicine Specialist and Associate Professor at the Hospital for Children (SickKids) and University of Toronto. Dr Toulany is also a health services researcher with advanced training in quality improvement. Her research focuses on quality of care for youth with chronic health conditions.

Kaveh Shojania, MD, is Vice Chair of Quality and Innovation in the Department of Medicine at the University of Toronto and a general internist at Sunnybrook Health Sciences Centre. His research focuses on patient safety and translating evidence into practice. From 2011 to 2020, Dr Shojania was Editor-in-Chief of BMJ Quality and Safety.

Creative Commons License

References

1. Berenson RA. If you can't measure performance, can you improve it? *JAMA*. 2016; 315(7): 645–46. https://doi.org/10.1001/jama.2016.0767.

2. Demming WE. *The new economics for industry, government, education*, 3rd ed. Cambridge, MA: MIT Press; 2018.

3. Martin GP, Aveling EL, Campbell A et al. Making soft intelligence hard: A multi-site qualitative study of challenges relating to voice about safety concerns. *BMJ Qual Saf*. 2018; 27: 710–717. https://doi.org/10.1136/bmjqs-2017-007579.

4. Martin GP, McKee L, Dixon-Woods M. Beyond metrics? Utilizing 'soft intelligence' for healthcare quality and safety. *Soc Sci Med*. 2015; 142: 19–26. https://doi.org/10.1016/j.socscimed.2015.07.027.

5. Donabedian A. Evaluating the quality of medical care. *Milbank Mem Fund Q*. 1966; 44(3): 166–206.

6. Donabedian A. The quality of care: How can it be assessed? *JAMA*. 1988; 260(12): 1743–48.

7. Donabedian A. *The definition of quality and approaches to its assessment*. Ann Arbor, MI: Health Administration Press; 1980.

8. Brook RH, McGlynn EA, Cleary PD. Measuring quality of care. *N Engl J Med*. 1996; 335(13): 966–70. https://doi.org/10.1056/nejm199609263351311.

9. Halm EA, Lee C, Chassin MR. Is volume related to outcome in health care? A systematic review and methodologic critique of the literature. *Ann Intern Med*. 2002; 137(6): 511–20. https://doi.org/10.7326/0003-4819-137-6-200209170-00012.

10. Birkmeyer JD, Siewers AE, Finlayson EV et al. Hospital volume and surgical mortality in the United States. *N Engl J Med*. 2002; 346(15): 1128–37. https://doi.org/10.1056/NEJMsa012337.

11. Birkmeyer JD, Stukel TA, Siewers AE et al. Surgeon volume and operative mortality in the United States. *N Engl J Med*. 2003; 349(22): 2117–27.

12. Meyer GS, Massagli MP. The forgotten component of the quality triad: Can we still learn something from 'structure'? *Jt Comm J Qual Improv*. 2001; 27 (9): 484–93.

13. Aiken LH, Clarke SP, Sloane DM, Sochalski J, Silber JH. Hospital nurse staffing and patient mortality, nurse burnout, and job dissatisfaction. *JAMA*. 2002; 288(16): 1987–93.

14. Shekelle PG. Nurse-patient ratios as a patient safety strategy: A systematic review. *Ann Intern Med.* 2013; 158(5 Pt 2): 404–409. https://doi.org/10.7326/0003-4819-158-5-201303051-00007.

15. Nallamothu BK, Normand SL, Wang Y et al. Relation between door-to-balloon times and mortality after primary percutaneous coronary intervention over time: A retrospective study. *Lancet.* 2015; 385(9973): 1114–22. https://doi.org/10.1016/s0140-6736(14)61932-2.

16. Kuhrij L, van Zwet E, van den Berg-Vos R, Nederkoorn P, Marang-van de Mheen PJ. Enhancing feedback on performance measures: The difference in outlier detection using a binary versus continuous outcome funnel plot and implications for quality improvement. *BMJ Qual Saf.* 2021; 30(1): 38–45. https://doi.org/10.1136/bmjqs-2019-009929.

17. Mant J, Hicks N. Detecting differences in quality of care: The sensitivity of measures of process and outcome in treating acute myocardial infarction. *BMJ.* 1995; 311(7008): 793–96.

18. Bradley EH, Herrin J, Wang Y et al. Strategies for reducing the door-to-balloon time in acute myocardial infarction. *N Engl J Med.* 2006; 355(22): 2308–20. https://doi.org/10.1056/NEJMsa063117.

19. Hofstede SN, Ceyisakar IE, Lingsma HF, Kringos DS, Marang-van de Mheen PJ. Ranking hospitals: Do we gain reliability by using composite rather than individual indicators? *BMJ Qual Saf.* 2019; 28: 94–102. https://doi.org/10.1136/bmjqs-2017-007669.

20. Varagunam M, Hutchings A, Black N. Do patient-reported outcomes offer a more sensitive method for comparing the outcomes of consultants than mortality? A multilevel analysis of routine data. *BMJ Qual Saf.* 2015; 24 (3): 195–202. https://doi.org/10.1136/bmjqs-2014-003551.

21. Iezzoni LI. 100 apples divided by 15 red herrings: A cautionary tale from the mid-19th century on comparing hospital mortality rates. *Ann Intern Med.* 1996; 124(12): 1079–85.

22. Shahian DM, Normand SL. What is a performance outlier? *BMJ Qual Saf.* 2015; 24(2): 95–99. https://doi.org/10.1136/bmjqs-2015-003934.

23. Shahian DM, Wolf RE, Iezzoni LI, Kirle L, Normand SL. Variability in the measurement of hospital-wide mortality rates. *N Engl J Med.* 2010; 363 (26): 2530–39. https://doi.org/10.1056/NEJMsa1006396.

24. Wadhera RK, Maddox KE Joynt, Wasfy JH et al. Association of the hospital readmissions reduction program with mortality among medicare beneficiaries hospitalized for heart failure, acute myocardial infarction, and pneumonia. *JAMA.* 2018; 320(24): 2542–52. https;//doi.org/10.1001/jama.2018.19232.

25. Gupta A, Allen LA, Bhatt DL et al. Association of the hospital readmissions reduction program implementation with readmission and mortality outcomes in heart failure. *JAMA Cardiol.* 2018; 3(1): 44–53. https://doi.org/10.1001/jamacardio.2017.4265.

26. Marang-van de Mheen PJ, Shojania KG. Simpson's paradox: How performance measurement can fail even with perfect risk adjustment. *BMJ Qual Saf.* 2014; 23(9): 701–705. https://doi.org/10.1136/bmjqs-2014-003358.

27. Shashikumar SA, Waken RJ, Luke AA, Nerenz DR, Maddox KE Joynt. Association of stratification by proportion of patients dually enrolled in medicare and medicaid with financial penalties in the hospital-acquired condition reduction program. *JAMA Intern Med.* 2021; 181(3): 330–38. https://doi.org/10.1001/jamainternmed.2020.7386.

28. Maddox KE Joynt, Reidhead M, Hu J et al. Adjusting for social risk factors impacts performance and penalties in the hospital readmissions reduction program. *Health Serv Res.* 2019; 54(2): 327–36. https://doi.org/10.1111/1475-6773.13133.

29. Zuckerman RB, Maddox KE Joynt, Sheingold SH, Chen LM, Epstein AM. Effect of a hospital-wide measure on the readmissions reduction program. *N Engl J Med.* 2017; 377(16): 1551–58. https://doi.org/10.1056/NEJMsa1701791.

30. Rajaram R, Chung JW, Kinnier CV et al. Hospital characteristics associated with penalties in the centers for medicare & medicaid services hospital-acquired condition reduction program. *JAMA.* 2015; 314(4): 375–83. https://doi.org/10.1001/jama.2015.8609.

31. Levtzion-Korach O, Frankel A, Alcalai H et al. Integrating incident data from five reporting systems to assess patient safety: Making sense of the elephant. *Jt Comm J Qual Patient Saf.* 2010; 36(9): 402–10. https://doi.org/10.1016/s1553-7250(10)36059-4.

32. Shojania KG. The elephant of patient safety: What you see depends on how you look. *Jt Comm J Qual Patient Saf.* 2010; 36(9): 399–401.

33. Reeves S, Kuper A, Hodges BD. Qualitative research methodologies: Ethnography. *BMJ.* 2008; 337: a1020. https://doi.org/10.1136/bmj.a1020.

34. Hor SY, Iedema R, Manias E. Creating spaces in intensive care for safe communication: A video-reflexive ethnographic study. *BMJ Qual Saf.* 2014; 23(12): 1007–13. https://doi.org/10.1136/bmjqs-2014-002835.

35. Liberati EG, Tarrant C, Willars J et al. Seven features of safety in maternity units: A framework based on multisite ethnography and stakeholder consultation. *BMJ Qual Saf.* 2021; 30: 444–56 https://doi.org/10.1136/bmjqs-2020-010988.

36. Manojlovich M, Frankel RM, Harrod M et al. Formative evaluation of the video reflexive ethnography method, as applied to the physician-nurse dyad. *BMJ Qual Saf.* 2019; 28(2): 160–66. https://doi.org/10.1136/bmjqs-2017-007728.

37. Tarrant C, Leslie M, Bion J, Dixon-Woods M. A qualitative study of speaking out about patient safety concerns in intensive care units. *Soc Sci Med.* 2017; 193: 8–15. https://doi.org/10.1016/j.socscimed.2017.09.036.

38. Dixon-Woods M, Bosk CL, Aveling EL, Goeschel CA, Pronovost PJ. Explaining michigan: Developing an ex post theory of a quality improvement program. *Milbank Q.* 2011; 89(2): 167–205. https://doi.org/10.1111/j.1468-0009.2011.00625.x.

39. Dixon-Woods M, Leslie M, Tarrant C, Bion J. Explaining matching Michigan: An ethnographic study of a patient safety program. *Implement Sci.* 2013; 8: 70. https://doi.org/10.1186/1748-5908-8-70.

40. Benning A, Ghaleb M, Suokas A et al. Large scale organisational intervention to improve patient safety in four UK hospitals: Mixed method evaluation. *BMJ.* 2011; 342: d195. https://doi.org/10.1136/bmj.d195.

41. Zamboni K, Singh S, Tyagi M et al. Effect of collaborative quality improvement on stillbirths, neonatal mortality and newborn care practices in hospitals of Telangana and Andhra Pradesh, India: Evidence from a quasi-experimental mixed-methods study. *Implement Sci.* 2021; 16(1): 4. https://doi.org/10.1186/s13012-020-01058-z.

42. Ling VB, Levi EE, Harrington AR et al. The cost of improving care: A multisite economic analysis of hospital resource use for implementing recommended postpartum contraception programmes. *BMJ Qual Saf.* 2021; 30: 658–67. https://doi.org/10.1136/bmjqs-2020-011111.

43. Shojania KG. Beyond clabsi and cauti: Broadening our vision of patient safety. *BMJ Qual Saf.* 2020; 29(5): 361–64. https://doi.org/10.1136/bmjqs-2019-010498.

44. Kwan JL, Lo L, Ferguson J et al. Computerised clinical decision support systems and absolute improvements in care: Meta-analysis of controlled clinical trials. *BMJ.* 2020; 370: m3216. https://doi.org/10.1136/bmj.m3216.

45. Woodcock T, Liberati EG, Dixon-Woods M. A mixed-methods study of challenges experienced by clinical teams in measuring improvement. *BMJ Qual Saf.* 2021; 30(2):106–15. https://doi.org/10.1136/bmjqs-2018-009048.

46. Davidoff F, Dixon-Woods M, Leviton L, Michie S. Demystifying theory and its use in improvement. *BMJ Qual Saf.* 2015; 24(3): 228–38. https://doi.org/10.1136/bmjqs-2014-003627.

47. Foy R, Ovretveit J., Shekelle PG et al. The role of theory in research to develop and evaluate the implementation of patient safety practices. *BMJ Qual Saf.* 2011; 20(5): 453–59. https://doi.org/10.1136/bmjqs.2010.047993.

48. Morris S, Ramsay AIG, Boaden RJ et al. Impact and sustainability of centralising acute stroke services in English metropolitan areas: Retrospective analysis of hospital episode statistics and stroke national audit data. *BMJ.* 2019; 364: 11. https://doi.org/10.1136/bmj.l1.

49. NHS. Hospital episode statistics (HES). https://digital.nhs.uk/data-and-information/data-tools-and-services/data-services/hospital-episode-statis tics. (Accessed 15 April 2024).

50. Cecil E, Bottle A, Esmail A et al. Investigating the association of alerts from a national mortality surveillance system with subsequent hospital mortality in England: An interrupted time series analysis. *BMJ Qual Saf.* 2018; 27(12): 965–73. https://doi.org/10.1136/bmjqs-2017-007495.

51. Reeson M, Forster A, van Walraven C. Incidence and trends of central line associated pneumothorax using radiograph report text search versus adminis- trative database codes. *BMJ Qual Saf.* 2018; 27(12): 982–88. https://doi.org/ 10.1136/bmjqs-2017-007715.

52. Gagalova KK, Elizalde MA Leon, Portales-Casamar E, Görges M. What you need to know before implementing a clinical research data ware- house: Comparative review of integrated data repositories in health care institutions. *JMIR Form Res.* 2020; 4(8): e17687. https://doi.org/10.2196/ 17687.

53. Pavlenko E, Strech D, Langhof H. Implementation of data access and use procedures in clinical data warehouses. A systematic review of literature and publicly available policies. *BMC Med Inform Decis Mak.* 2020; 20(1): 157. https://doi.org/10.1186/s12911-020-01177-z.

54. Murray SG, Yim JWL, Croci R et al. Using spatial and temporal mapping to identify nosocomial disease transmission of clostridium difficile. *JAMA Intern Med.* 2017; 177(12): 1863–65. https://doi.org/10.1001/jama internmed.2017.5506.

55. Gliklich RE, Dreyer NA, eds. *Registries for evaluating patient outcomes: A user's guide.* 2nd ed. AHRQ publication no.10-ehc049. Rockville, MD: Agency for healthcare research and quality. September 2010.

56. Hall BL, Hamilton BH, Richards K et al. Does surgical quality improve in the American college of surgeons national surgical quality improvement program: An evaluation of all participating hospitals. *Ann Surg.* 2009; 250 (3): 363–76. https://doi.org/10.1097/SLA.0b013e3181b4148f.

57. Thakker A, Briggs N, Maeda A et al. Reducing the rate of post-surgical urinary tract infections in orthopedic patients. *BMJ Open Qual*. 2018; 7(2): e000177. https://doi.org/10.1136/bmjoq-2017-000177.

58. Quon BS, Goss CH. A story of success: Continuous quality improvement in cystic fibrosis care in the USA. *Thorax*. 2011; 66(12): 1106–108. https://doi.org/10.1136/thoraxjnl-2011-200611.

59. Ludvigsson JF, Andersson M, Bengtsson J et al. Swedish inflammatory bowel disease register (SWIBREG) – a nationwide quality register. *Scand J Gastroenterol*. 2019; 54(9): 1089–101. https://doi.org/10.1080/0036 5521.2019.1660799.

60. Castro M, Papadatou B, Baldassare M et al. Inflammatory bowel disease in children and adolescents in Italy: Data from the pediatric national IBD register (1996–2003). *Inflamm Bowel Dis*. 2008; 14(9): 1246–52. https://doi.org/10.1002/ibd.20470.

61. Baines R, Langelaan M, de Bruijne M, Spreeuwenberg P, Wagner C. How effective are patient safety initiatives? A retrospective patient record review study of changes to patient safety over time. *BMJ Qual Saf*. 2015; 24(9): 561–71. https://doi.org/10.1136/bmjqs-2014-003702.

62. Landrigan CP, Parry GJ, Bones CB et al. Temporal trends in rates of patient harm resulting from medical care. *N Engl J Med*. 2010; 363(22): 2124–34. https://doi.org/10.1056/NEJMsa1004404.

63. Seng EC, Mehdipour S, Simpson S, Gabriel RA. Tracking persistent postoperative opioid use: A proof-of-concept study demonstrating a use case for natural language processing. *Reg Anesth Pain Med*. 2024; 49: 241–47. https://doi.org/10.1136/rapm-2023-104629.

64. Wang L, Zhang Y, Chignell M et al. Boosting delirium identification accuracy with sentiment-based natural language processing: Mixed methods study. *JMIR Med Inform*. 2022; 10(12): e38161. https://doi.org/10.2196/38161.

65. Starmer AJ, Spector ND, Srivastava R et al. Changes in medical errors after implementation of a handoff program. *N Engl J Med*. 2014; 371(19): 1803–12. https://doi.org/10.1056/NEJMsa1405556.

66. Stockwell DC, Bisarya H, Classen DC et al. A trigger tool to detect harm in pediatric inpatient settings. *Pediatrics*. 2015; 135(6): 1036–42. https://doi.org/10.1542/peds.2014-2152.

67. Matlow AG, Baker GR, Flintoft V et al. Adverse events among children in Canadian hospitals: The Canadian paediatric adverse events study. *CMAJ*. 2012; 184(13): E709–18. https://doi.org/10.1503/cmaj.112153.

68. Hogan H, Zipfel R, Neuburger J et al. Avoidability of hospital deaths and association with hospital-wide mortality ratios: Retrospective case record review and regression analysis. *BMJ*. 2015; 351: h3239. https://doi.org/10.1136/bmj.h3239.

69. Mays N, Pope C. Qualitative research in health care: Assessing quality in qualitative research. *BMJ*. 2000; 320(7226): 50–52. https://doi.org/10.1136/bmj.320.7226.50.

70. Langford AV, Gnjidic D, Lin CC et al. Challenges of opioid deprescribing and factors to be considered in the development of opioid deprescribing guidelines: A qualitative analysis. *BMJ Qual Saf*. 2021; 30(2): 133–40. https://doi.org/10.1136/bmjqs-2020-010881.

71. Tarrant C, O'Donnell B, Martin G et al. A complex endeavour: An ethnographic study of the implementation of the sepsis six clinical care bundle. *Implement Sci*. 2016; 11(1): 149. https://doi.org/10.1186/s13012-016-0518-z.

72. Dixon-Woods M, Shaw RL, Agarwal S, Smith JA. The problem of appraising qualitative research. *Qual Saf Health Care*. 2004; 13(3): 223–25. https://doi.org/10.1136/qhc.13.3.223.

73. Robert G, Cornwell J, Black N. Friends and family test should no longer be mandatory. *BMJ*. 2018; 360: k367. https://doi.org/10.1136/bmj.k367.

74. Davidson KW, Shaffer J, Ye S et al. Interventions to improve hospital patient satisfaction with healthcare providers and systems: A systematic review. *BMJ Qual Saf*. 2017; 26(7): 596–606. https://doi.org/10.1136/bmjqs-2015-004758.

75. Hedges C, Hunt C, Ball P. Quiet time improves the patient experience. *J Nurs Care Qual*. 2019; 34(3): 197–202. https://doi.org/10.1097/ncq.0000000000000363.

76. Griffiths A, Leaver MP. Wisdom of patients: Predicting the quality of care using aggregated patient feedback. *BMJ Qual Saf*. 2018; 27(2): 110–18. https://doi.org/10.1136/bmjqs-2017-006847.

77. Etchells E, Trbovich P. Five golden rules for successful measurement of improvement. *BMJ Qual Saf*. 2023; 32(10): 566–69. https://doi.org/10.1136/bmjqs-2023-016129.

78. McGuckin M, Govednik J. Patient empowerment and hand hygiene, 1997–2012. *J Hosp Infect*. 2013; 84(3): 191–99. https://doi.org/10.1016/j.jhin.2013.01.014.

79. Gordon SC. A piece of my mind: Ask me if I cleaned my hands. *JAMA*. 2012; 307(15): 1591–92. https://doi.org/10.1001/jama.2012.474.

80. Bosk CL, Dixon-Woods M, Goeschel CA, Pronovost PJ. Reality check for checklists. *Lancet*. 2009; 374(9688): 444–45. https://doi.org/10.1016/s0140-6736(09)61440-9.

81. Weller JM, Jowsey T, Skilton C et al. Improving the quality of administration of the surgical safety checklist: A mixed methods study in New Zealand hospitals. *BMJ Open*. 2018; 8(12): e022882. https://doi.org/10.1136/bmjopen-2018-022882.

82. Vats A, Vincent CA, Nagpal K et al. Practical challenges of introducing WHO surgical checklist: UK pilot experience. *BMJ*. 2010; 340: b5433. https://doi.org/10.1136/bmj.b5433.

83. Davies SM, Geppert J, McClellan M et al. AHRQ technical reviews. *Refinement of the HCUP quality indicators*. Rockville, MD: Agency for Healthcare Research and Quality; 2001.

84. Shojania KG, Forster AJ. Hospital mortality: When failure is not a good measure of success. *CMAJ*. 2008; 179(2): 153–57. https://doi.org/10.1503/cmaj.080010.

85. Greaves F, Ramirez-Cano D, Millett C, Darzi A, Donaldson L. Harnessing the cloud of patient experience: Using social media to detect poor quality healthcare. *BMJ Qual Saf*. 2013; 22(3): 251–55. https://doi.org/10.1136/bmjqs-2012-001527.

86. Meyer GS, Massagli MP. The forgotten component of the quality triad: Can we still learn something from 'structure'? *Jt Comm J Qual Improv*. 2001; 27 (9): 484–93. https://doi.org/10.1016/s1070-3241(01)27042-4.

87. Tsai TC, Joynt KE, Orav EJ, Gawande AA, Jha AK. Variation in surgical-readmission rates and quality of hospital care. *N Engl J Med*. 2013; 369 (12): 1134–42. https://doi.org/10.1056/NEJMsa1303118.

88. Dimick JB, Ghaferi AA. Hospital readmission as a quality measure in surgery. *JAMA*. 2015; 313(5): 512–13. https://doi.org/10.1001/jama.2014.14179.

89. Mangione-Smith R, DeCristofaro AH, Setodji CM et al. The quality of ambulatory care delivered to children in the United States. *N Engl J Med*. 2007; 357(15): 1515–23. https://doi.org/10.1056/NEJMsa064637.

90. McGlynn EA, Asch SM, Adams J et al. The quality of health care delivered to adults in the United States. *N Engl J Med*. 2003; 348(26): 2635–45. https://doi.org/10.1056/NEJMsa022615.

91. Tricco AC, Ivers NM, Grimshaw JM et al. Effectiveness of quality improvement strategies on the management of diabetes: A systematic review and meta-analysis. *Lancet*. 2012; 379(9833): 2252–61. https://doi.org/10.1016/s0140-6736(12)60480-2.

92. Lawthers AG, McCarthy EP, Davis RB et al. Identification of in-hospital complications from claims data. Is it valid? *Med Care*. 2000; 38(8): 785–95. https://doi.org/10.1097/00005650-200008000-00003.

93. Winters BD, Bharmal A, Wilson RF et al. Validity of the agency for health care research and quality patient safety indicators and the centers for medicare and medicaid hospital-acquired conditions: A systematic review and meta-analysis. *Med Care*. 2016; 54(12): 1105–11. https://doi.org/10.1097/mlr.0000000000000550.

94. Lilford R, Pronovost P. Using hospital mortality rates to judge hospital performance: A bad idea that just won't go away. *BMJ*. 2010; 340: c2016. https://doi.org/10.1136/bmj.c2016.

95. Shojania KG, Forster AJ. Hospital mortality: When failure is not a good measure of success. *CMAJ*. 2008; 179(2): 153–57. https://doi.org/10.1503/cmaj.080010.

96. Hayward RA, Hofer TP. Estimating hospital deaths due to medical errors: Preventability is in the eye of the reviewer. *JAMA*. 2001; 286(4): 415–20.

97. Hodgson K, Deeny SR, Steventon A. Ambulatory care-sensitive conditions: Their potential uses and limitations. *BMJ Qual Saf*. 2019; 28(6): 429–33. https://doi.org/10.1136/bmjqs-2018-008820.

98. Billings J, Zeitel L, Lukomnik J et al. Impact of socioeconomic status on hospital use in New York City. *Health Aff*. 1993; 12(1): 162–73. https://doi.org/10.1377/hlthaff.12.1.162.

99. Lynch B, Fitzgerald AP, Corcoran P et al. Drivers of potentially avoidable emergency admissions in Ireland: An ecological analysis. *BMJ Qual Saf*. 2019; 28(6): 438–48. https://doi.org/10.1136/bmjqs-2018-008002.

100. Bettenhausen JL, Colvin JD, Berry JG et al. Association of income inequality with pediatric hospitalizations for ambulatory care-sensitive conditions. *JAMA Pediatr*. 2017; 171(6): e170322. https://doi.org/10.1001/jamapediatrics.2017.0322.

101. Goldfeld S, Paton K, Lei S, Perera P, Hiscock H. Trends in rates and inequalities in paediatric admissions for ambulatory care sensitive conditions in Victoria, Australia (2003 to 2013). *J Paediatr Child Health*. 2021; 57: 860–66. https://doi.org/10.1111/jpc.15338.

102. Lumme S, Manderbacka K, Arffman M, Karvonen S, Keskimaki I. Cumulative social disadvantage and hospitalisations due to ambulatory care-sensitive conditions in Finland in 2011–2013: A register study. *BMJ Open*. 2020; 10(8): e038338. https://doi.org/10.1136/bmjopen-2020-038338.

103. Agency for Healthcare Research and Quality. Patient safety indicator 08 (PSI 08) in hospital fall with hip fracture rate. Rockville: 2017. https://qualityindicators.ahrq.gov/Downloads/Modules/PSI/V60-ICD09/TechSpecs/PSI_08_In_Hospital_Fall_with_Hip_Fracture_Rate.pdf (accessed 16 April 2024).

104. Dixon-Woods M, Leslie M, Bion J, Tarrant C. What counts? An ethnographic study of infection data reported to a patient safety program. *Milbank Q*. 2012; 90(3): 548–91. https://doi.org/10.1111/j.1468-0009.2012.00674.x.

105. Etchells E, Ho M, Shojania KG. Value of small sample sizes in rapid-cycle quality improvement projects. *BMJ Qual Saf.* 2016; 25(3): 202–206. https://doi.org/10.1136/bmjqs-2015-005094.

106. Craig SL, Feinstein AR. Antecedent therapy versus detection bias as causes of neoplastic multimorbidity. *Am J Clin Oncol.* 1999; 22(1): 51–56. https://doi.org/10.1097/00000421-199902000-00013.

107. Haut ER, Pronovost PJ. Surveillance bias in outcomes reporting. *JAMA.* 2011; 305(23): 2462–63. https://doi.org/10.1001/jama.2011.822.

108. Bilimoria KY, Chung J, Ju MH et al. Evaluation of surveillance bias and the validity of the venous thromboembolism quality measure. *JAMA.* 2013; 310(14): 1482–89. https://doi.org/10.1001/jama.2013.280048.

109. Decker SG Van, Bosch N, Murphy J. Catheter-associated urinary tract infection reduction in critical care units: A bundled care model. *BMJ Open Qual.* 2021; 10(4): e001534. https://doi.org/10.1136/bmjoq-2021-001534.

110. Vaughn VM, Chopra V. Revisiting the panculture. *BMJ Qual Saf.* 2017; 26 (3): 236–39. https://doi.org/10.1136/bmjqs-2015-004821.

111. Mullin KM, Kovacs CS, Fatica C et al. A multifaceted approach to reduction of catheter-associated urinary tract infections in the intensive care unit with an emphasis on 'stewardship of culturing'. *Infect Control Hosp Epidemiol.* 2017; 38(2): 186–88. https://doi.org/10.1017/ice.2016.266.

112. Hawkins JB, Brownstein JS, Tuli G et al. Measuring patient-perceived quality of care in US hospitals using Twitter. *BMJ Qual Saf.* 2016; 25: 404–13. https://doi.org/10.1136/bmjqs-2015-004309.

113. Sewalk KC, Tuli G, Hswen Y, Brownstein JS, Hawkins JB. Using Twitter to examine web-based patient experience sentiments in the United States: Longitudinal study. *J Med Internet Res.* 2018; 20(10): e10043. https://doi.org/10.2196/10043.

114. Hotchkiss RS, Moldawer LL, Opal SM et al. Sepsis and septic shock. *Nat Rev Dis Primers.* 2016; 2: 16045. https://doi.org/10.1038/nrdp.2016.45.

115. Gupta RG, Hartigan SM, Kashiouris MG, Sessler CN, Bearman GM. Early goal-directed resuscitation of patients with septic shock: Current evidence and future directions. *Crit Care.* 2015; 19(1): 286. https://doi.org/10.1186/s13054-015-1011-9.

116. Shojania KG. Incident reporting systems: What will it take to make them less frustrating and achieve anything useful? *Jt Comm J Qual Patient Saf.* 2021; 47(12): 755–58. https://doi.org/10.1016/j.jcjq.2021.10.001.

117. Barker AL, Morello RT, Wolfe R et al. 6-pack programme to decrease fall injuries in acute hospitals: Cluster randomised controlled trial. *BMJ.* 2016; 352: h6781. https://doi.org/10.1136/bmj.h6781.

118. Dykes PC, Burns Z, Adelman J et al. Evaluation of a patient-centered fall-prevention tool kit to reduce falls and injuries: A nonrandomized controlled trial. *JAMA Netw Open*. 2020; 3(11): e2025889. https://doi.org/10.1001/jamanetworkopen.2020.25889.

119. Shojania KG. The frustrating case of incident-reporting systems. *Qual Saf Health Care*. 2008; 17(6): 400–402. https://doi.org/10.1136/qshc.2008.029496.

120. Liberman AL, Newman-Toker DE. Symptom-disease pair analysis of diagnostic error (spade): A conceptual framework and methodological approach for unearthing misdiagnosis-related harms using big data. *BMJ Qual Saf*. 2018; 27(7): 557–66. https://doi.org/10.1136/bmjqs-2017-007032.

121. Adelman JS, Applebaum JR, Schechter CB et al. Effect of restriction of the number of concurrently open records in an electronic health record on wrong-patient order errors: A randomized clinical trial. *JAMA*. 2019; 321 (18): 1780–87. https://doi.org/10.1001/jama.2019.3698.

122. Adelman JS, Kalkut GE, Schechter CB et al. Understanding and preventing wrong-patient electronic orders: A randomized controlled trial. *J Am Med Inform Assoc*. 2013; 20(2): 305–10. https://doi.org/10.1136/amiajnl-2012-001055.

123. Ocloo J, Matthews R. From tokenism to empowerment: Progressing patient and public involvement in healthcare improvement. *BMJ Qual Saf*. 2016; 25(8): 626–32. https://doi.org/10.1136/bmjqs-2015-004839.

124. Batalden PB, Davidoff F. What is 'quality improvement' and how can it transform healthcare? *Qual Saf Health Care*. 2007; 16(1): 2–3. https://doi.org/10.1136/qshc.2006.022046.

125. Berwick DM. Controlling variation in health care: A consultation from Walter Shewhart. *Med Care*. 1991; 29(12): 1212–25. https://doi.org/10.1097/00005650-199112000-00004.

126. Berwick DM. A primer on leading the improvement of systems. *BMJ*. 1996; 312(7031): 619–22. https://doi.org/10.1136/bmj.312.7031.619.

127. Best M, Neuhauser D. Shewhart Walter A, 1924, and the Hawthorne factory. *Qual Saf Health Care*. 2006; 15(2): 142–43. https://doi.org/10.1136/qshc.2006.018093.

128. Langley GJ, Moen RD, Nolan KM, Nolan TW, Norman CL, Provost LP. *The improvement guide: A practical approach to enhancing organizational performance*. San Francisco, CA: Jossey-Bass; 2009.

129. Provost L, Murray S. *The health care data guide: Learning from data for improvement*. San Francisco, CA: Jossey-Bass; 2011.

Cambridge Elements ☰

Improving Quality and Safety in Healthcare

Editors-in-Chief

Mary Dixon-Woods

THIS Institute (The Healthcare Improvement Studies Institute)

Mary is Director of THIS Institute and is the Health Foundation Professor of Healthcare Improvement Studies in the Department of Public Health and Primary Care at the University of Cambridge. Mary leads a programme of research focused on healthcare improvement, healthcare ethics, and methodological innovation in studying healthcare.

Graham Martin

THIS Institute (The Healthcare Improvement Studies Institute)

Graham is Director of Research at THIS Institute, leading applied research programmes and contributing to the institute's strategy and development. His research interests are in the organisation and delivery of healthcare, and particularly the role of professionals, managers, and patients and the public in efforts at organisational change.

Executive Editor

Katrina Brown

THIS Institute (The Healthcare Improvement Studies Institute)

Katrina was Communications Manager at THIS Institute, providing editorial expertise to maximise the impact of THIS Institute's research findings. She managed the project to produce the series until 2023.

Editorial Team

Sonja Marjanovic

RAND Europe

Sonja is Director of RAND Europe's healthcare innovation, industry, and policy research. Her work provides decision-makers with evidence and insights to support innovation and improvement in healthcare systems, and to support the translation of innovation into societal benefits for healthcare services and population health.

Tom Ling

RAND Europe

Tom is Head of Evaluation at RAND Europe and President of the European Evaluation Society, leading evaluations and applied research focused on the key challenges facing health services. His current health portfolio includes evaluations of the innovation landscape, quality improvement, communities of practice, patient flow, and service transformation.

Ellen Perry

THIS Institute (The Healthcare Improvement Studies Institute)

Ellen supported the production of the series during 2020–21.

Gemma Petley

THIS Institute (The Healthcare Improvement Studies Institute)

Gemma is Senior Communications and Editorial Manager at THIS Institute, responsible for overseeing the production and maximising the impact of the series.

Claire Dipple

THIS Institute (The Healthcare Improvement Studies Institute)

Claire is Editorial Project Manager at THIS Institute, responsible for editing and project managing the series.

About the Series

The past decade has seen enormous growth in both activity and research on improvement in healthcare. This series offers a comprehensive and authoritative set of overviews of the different improvement approaches available, exploring the thinking behind them, examining evidence for each approach, and identifying areas of debate.

Cambridge Elements ≡

Improving Quality and Safety in Healthcare

Elements in the Series

Printed in the United States
by Baker & Taylor Publisher Services